SHILAJIT:
A NATURAL HEALER

A Beginner's Guide to Shilajit

Dr. Zainab Sikander

DEDICATION

To all my
valuable readers!

TABLE OF CONTENTS

INTRODUCTION

Before the discovery of pharmaceutical interventions and the latest methods for the treatment and prevention of diseases, people were relying on remedies that were provided by the nature. People from the past used natural therapeutic medicines to treat wounds, fever, fatigue, headaches, and stomach problems. Even for the serious disorder, the only source of relief was medicines derived from herbs, plants, animals, minerals, rocks, and other natural sources. Among them, there was a unique material with an ultimate therapeutic profile and an abundance of active molecules. This dark-colored material is secreted by the layers of the mountain located at high altitudes such as the Himalayas and is formed by the gradual decomposition of plants, animals, and other minerals. This unique blackish material is known as Shilajit. Shilajit was initially used in traditional medicine about 4000 years ago, and it is still termed an integral part of Ayurvedic medicine.

Shilajit is a potent dietary supplement that has high nutritional value and is a safer option as compared to other pharmaceutically or chemically synthesized supplements. It is known for its extraordinary healing and curative powers that can help to cope with a large number of diseases known to man. From acute to chronic and mild to severe health concerns including indigestion, hypertension, cramps, fatigue, general weakness, cancer, diabetes, Alzheimer's, anemia, and depression, shilajit proves itself as the best nutraceutical. In addition to the magical healing skills of shilajit, its ability to boost energy, fight internal and external health destroyers, and improve the standard of living is also inevitable. Moreover, the use of shilajit as a workout supplement further increases its value.

In a nutshell, there are a lot of other interesting and useful facts regarding the shilajit that you should know if you really care about your and your loved ones' health. Regarding shilajit, there are a lot

of information resources available online and offline that might confuse you and you might wonder if the info is authentic or is just someone's personal experience. But the good news, in the book "SHILAJIT: A Natural Healer", all minor and major details relevant to shilajit are extracted from reputed sources. For the book, each and every detail is acquired from journals, articles, and books that are approved by health experts and are highly acclaimed. In this book, all the basic and important features of shilajit are explained in detail, including:

- Origin of shilajit

- History

- Types

- Composition

- Mechanism of action

- Methods of purification

- Medicinal properties

- Benefits for physical health

- Benefits for mental health

- Uses in specific diseases

- Complimentary role to other therapies

- Potential side effects

- Required dosages

And many more!

Therefore, this book is a must-read, whether you are newly introduced to this magical herb or are a pro and already have extensive knowledge. This book comes in handy in every situation and can help you to easily understand shilajit and its healing properties through the plain and simple language used. Thus, you are highly recommended to give this book a try and you will eventually understand that the book **"SHILAJIT: A Natural Healer"** is worth reading as it unveils the virtues of the miraculous natural healer, known as SHILAJIT.

CHAPTER #1
INTRODUCTION TO SHILAJIT

Shilajit is a natural substance that has a sticky-tar-like consistency and is blackish-brown in color. It is formed by the slow decomposition of certain plants and minerals at high altitudes, approximately 1000 to 5000 meters above sea level, and is found mainly in the mountains of the Himalayas between India and Nepal. Shilajit was initially used in Ayurvedic Medicine due to its potential healing properties and still now, people use it as a dietary supplement for protection against diseases and to improve their lifestyle.

The healing and therapeutic characteristics of Shilajit are dependent on the region from which it is extracted. Moreover, it is known by different names and the most common English names used are Mineral pitch and Asphaltum. Other names for Shilajit include Salajit, Shilajatu, Silajatu, Moomie, Moomiyo, and Andean Shilajit.

WHICH COUNTRIES PRODUCE SHILAJIT?

Shilajit is a natural supplement that has a high nutritional and medicinal profile and is mainly found in the mountains of the Himalayas. Besides the Himalayas, shilajit extracts are also present in Altai Mountain and the Karakoram. Other countries that are rich in the natural deposits of shilajit include North Chile, Russia, Pakistan, India, Tibet, Nepal, Afghanistan, Bhutan, Iran, Mongolia, and Central Asia.

HOW SHILAJIT IS FORMED?

The formation of Shilajit is not a matter of days. Instead, it takes years to produce Shilajit from the gradual decomposition of plants and minerals. Regarding the formation of Shilajit, there are several theories that explain how Shilajit is produced from certain raw materials. According to Tibetan and Ayurvedic experts, Shilajit is produced from the melting of metals like iron, copper, gold, and silver. Another group of scholars proposed that Shilajit is obtained from the gradual decomposition of marine animals and certain plants including Trifolium repens, Euphorbia royleana, Dumortiera, Minium, Plagiochasma, and many other higher plants. Another group of experts believed that Shilajit is derived from urine and fecal content of specific birds, squirrels, and other animals, and the secretions of certain plants.

The theory of slow decomposition of plants and minerals is more acceptable and according to several studies, during the process of decomposition, the organic matter of decaying content undergoes a series of changes. These changes take place under high temperatures and pressure and involve the transformation of humic acid into natural gas and residual carbon. In the summer days, the mountains get warm, due to which, the by-product of decomposition, Shilajit, becomes viscous and starts oozing out from the cracks of the rock. Here, people collect it by hand and send it over for purification.

PURIFICATION OF SHILAJIT

The purification of shilajit is extremely important because shilajit, in its raw form obtained from rocks, has impurities that make it unsuitable for human consumption. Moreover, these impurities will also lower the therapeutic and healing powers. Thus, after obtaining from mountains, shilajit is subjected to a series of purifying steps that will enhance its curative strength. Usually, four methods are used for the purification of shilajit.

1) Triphala Decoction

Triphala decoction, also known as Dashmool Decoction, is the most common technique used for the purification of shilajit. This method will provide pure Shilajit that will have additional curative powers due to the presence of medicinal herbs. This technique takes 3 to 4 days to complete and is consist of the following steps:

- Mix Triphala powder with water in a ratio of 1:6 respectively, and prepare a mixture in an iron pot.

- Now, cook this mixture on the stove on a low flame and let it boil.

- When the mixture reduces to ¼ of the total quantity, remove it from the stove and filter this Triphala solution.

- Now, transfer the prepared Triphala mixture to a large bowl and add 1500 grams of shilajit pieces to the same bowl.

- Now, let shilajit soak in the Triphala decoction for 24 hours. After that, put the mixture on the stove for reheating.

- Due to heating, shilajit will begin to dissolve and start floating on the surface of the mixture. Separate the shilajit from the surface.

- Now, heat the shilajit, separated from the mixture, on a low flame to remove any excess fluid. Keep on heating until the solution becomes thicker.

- Now, turn off the flame and let it dry under the sun.

- The final product will be in powder form having greyish color and is bitter in taste.

2) Altai Method

The Altai method is a lengthy and difficult procedure but this method provides pure shilajit with excellent nutritional and curative benefits. The Altai method consists of the following steps:

- Place raw shilajit in the particular container and put that container in cold water to harden the Shilajit.

- After the hardening of the shilajit, cut its top layer and place it again inside the container. Now, place the container in a water bath for an hour. This will evaporate the moisture and an oily solution will be left behind. Collect this oily solution.

- Now, cool down the collected oily solution at room temperature. Within 2 weeks, shilajit begins to rise on the surface and forms a separate layer.

- The shilajit formed is then collected from the surface and is free from impurities.

- Now, spread the beeswax on the wooden tray and pour the collected shilajit on the tray.

- Place the trays in the open air to remove moisture and cover them with gauze.

3) Thermal Evaporation

The thermal evaporation technique is the most efficient, time-saving, and pocket-friendly method for the easy purification of raw shilajit. Through evaporation, a large quantity of shilajit can be purified easily in a shorter time. But this method could potentially affect the healing profile of Shilajit and it may lose its potency and effectiveness. Thermal evaporation involves the following steps:

- The process begins by mixing raw shilajit in water and preparing a mixture that has a uniform consistency.

- Now, filter the solution and remove all the impurities or contaminants.

- The purified shilajit obtained is subjected to high temperature, preferably between 80°C - 90°C, to evaporate the water.

4)Centrifugation

Centrifugation is the oldest method used to purify and extract high-quality shilajit. The important steps involved in this method are:

- The centrifugation method uses a device, called a centrifuge.

- The centrifuge uses centrifugal force that works by separating the impurities and contaminants from the shilajit and producing pure shilajit products. There is no use of heat in the centrifugation method and thus, there will be no reduction in the healing and nutritional properties of shilajit.

PHYSICAL PROPERTIES OF SHILAJIT

In raw form, shilajit is a gooey, tar-like substance that has varying viscosity. The physical appearance of shilajit also depends upon the area from where it is collected. It is usually black or dark brown in color and it may also have a lighter color or have shades of red or amber color according to the region of its extraction.

COMPOSITION OF SHILAJIT

Shilajit comprises 60-80% organic content, 20-40% mineral content, and 5% of trace elements. The major component of Shilajit is humic substances that include humic acid, humans, and fulvic acid while it also contains 80 other bioactive elements including albuminoids, gums, fatty acids, benzoic acids, and resin. The humic content of Shilajit is obtained from the breakdown of organic matter and the healing characteristic of shilajit is mainly due to the presence of fulvic acid. Fulvic acid is water soluble and has a low molecular weight, that's why it has good absorption rates in the intestine and is excreted from the body within a few hours. Shilajit is also known as a Phyto-complex which means it contains both active and inactive molecules that are found in plants, and exhibit powerful antioxidant properties. It is believed that the chemical composition of shilajit is in accordance with the region of its formation and extraction, and on the basis of this, shilajit is also found to contain sterols, ichthyol, carboxylic acids, triterpenes, calcium, copper, manganese, zinc, selenium, phosphorus, lithium, iron, amino acids, and metabolites.

BENEFITS OF SHILAJIT

Shilajit offers countless health benefits and some of which include:

- Shilajit is well-known for its role in improving brain function by preventing cognitive diseases. It is often used in the treatment of Alzheimer's disease

- It is one of the best antiaging supplements that rejuvenates skin and keeps it healthy

- Shilajit is also used as an antidiabetic supplement

- It can aid in weight loss and prevent obesity

- It can increase the levels of the male sex hormone 'testosterone'

- It can improve cardiovascular health and prevent heart problems

- It exhibits strong antioxidant, anti-inflammatory, antihypertensive, and antiseptic properties

Besides, there are many other medicinal benefits of shilajit that are given in detail in the upcoming chapters.

CONCLUSIONS

Shilajit is an extremely useful natural substance that is widely used as a dietary supplement and is safe to use. It can help in the prevention of a number of diseases ranging from mild to moderate and even severe ones such as Alzheimer's. Not only for prevention and treatment but people also use shilajit to improve their overall health. In short, shilajit is a nutraceutical with innumerable health benefits. Owing to these amazing characteristics of shilajit, a lot of research has been done every year to figure out its effectiveness and to further explore its curative advantages in medical sciences, particularly in the neurological field. And medical experts believe that shilajit can shape the world of therapeutic science with its peculiar and extremely beneficial properties and this is the reason, why shilajit is extensively studied at the cellular as well as molecular level.

CHAPTER #2
HISTORY OF SHILAJIT

Shilajit is dark colored, blackish-brown material that has varying consistency and is distributed in several mountain ranges, especially in the Himalayas. It is composed of humic substances along with other important bioactive elements and nutrients and because of its versatile composition, shilajit is a favorite nutraceutical around the world.

In traditional medicine, shilajit is used for optimal brain functioning, as an antioxidant, as a therapeutic agent for rejuvenation, and for various other curative purposes. The majority of these medicinal properties of shilajit are confirmed by the latest medical studies and thus, its use is still in practice in various countries.

ORIGIN OF SHILAJIT

Shilajit is known to have its origin in the East where, in ancient days, Indians and people from other cultures use shilajit as a potent healing agent for a number of health issues. Known by the names of shilajit, shilajit, and memiya, it is produced by the slow decay of plants and minerals at high altitudes in the mountain ranges. Shilajit was mentioned in the writings of Avicenna, Paracleus, Al Buruni, and other well-known scholars, scientists, and philosophers indicating that shilajit was the oldest known natural healer. There are mixed estimates regarding the initial use of shilajit. According to some reports, the practice of shilajit was as old as 3000 years while other older records claimed that shilajit was first introduced approximately 5000 years in Indian culture and the Himalayan Mountains. That's why it was believed that shilajit originates from the mountain range of the Himalayas. Even today, the high-quality Shilajit is extracted from the Himalayan mountains and the Altai mountains, and both of these mountains are estimated to be 300 to 500 million years old.

In the Altai Mountain and other Eurasian Mountain ranges, another material similar to shilajit was discovered by the native people. This substance was named Moomiyo or Moomie and it was slightly different from shilajit in terms of chemical composition, potency, and time of discovery. But now, Moomiyo and Shilajit are viewed as different names for the same thing because they share similar physical and chemical characteristics.

A brief overview of the origin of shilajit is given below:

➢ **Shilajit in East**

Due to its immense popularity in the East, people began trading shilajit and eventually brought it to Europe. In Europe, shilajit received a welcoming response from kings and rulers due to its miraculous healing benefits. It became a highly valuable natural healer but was too expensive for everyone to buy. Only wealthy people were able to afford it and thus, it was viewed as a luxury item.

➢ Shilajit in West

Meanwhile, in the West, shilajit was first mentioned about 2500 years ago by the Greek philosopher, Aristotle. He elaborated the healing characteristics of Moomie and also pointed out the methods to find out the best quality of shilajit. Thus, it was concluded that shilajit was an important part of west culture from the very beginning.

➢ Shilajit in Modern times

In the late 1800 century, the shilajit was 'rediscovered' by a British explorer, Sir Martin E. Stanley and this discovery led to experiments and clinical trials on further exploring the therapeutic benefits of shilajit. Sir Martin Stanley observed that monkeys residing in the Himalayan mountains were active and looked younger even in their old age as compared to those that were living in Europe. On investigation, it was found that Himalayan monkeys were eating shilajit, a blackish tar-like material secreted by rocks and it was the reason for their agility and good health even in older age. After this amazing discovery, shilajit was reintroduced and a lot of research work and clinical trials were done to further explore its nutritional profile and to extract the maximum benefits. Moreover, people started looking for more reservoirs and this leads to the discovery of different forms of the shilajit in other mountain ranges of South America, Norway, and Africa.

HISTORY OF SHILAJIT USE IN AYURVEDIC MEDICINE

In today's world, we are constantly bombarded with information that can be difficult to process. With so many different voices speaking at once, it can be hard to cut through the static and discover what is fact and what is fiction. Fortunately, it is not difficult to find legitimate resources for learning about old and complex topics like Ayurvedic and Shilajit. In this chapter, all the information and details are obtained from trustworthy resources gathered from books, peer-reviewed journals, and other authentic articles that will answer your all questions like what is Ayurvedic medicine? How it is related to Shilajit? What are their history and uses? Thus, your all concerns are addressed here thoroughly which will not only educate you but will also save your precious time. Now, let's move toward the main subject, that is, how the use of shilajit is related to ayurvedic medicine. But before going deep into this, you should have sound knowledge of ayurvedic, its history, and why it is an important element of present living.

AYURVEDIC MEDICINE

Ayurvedic medicine is one of the oldest systems of medicine in the world, with clear records of its existence dating back to 5000 BC. Today, this discipline is still very popular and gained popularity for its holistic approach to wellness and prevention through diet and lifestyle interventions.

Ayurvedic medicine is a holistic practice that has its origins in India. It's also known as "the science of life" because it emphasizes on the balance between different energies to treat individual needs. There are several parameters that define ayurvedic practice and set it apart from other traditional practices dealing with wellness and prevention.

Ayurvedic medicine or simply, Ayurveda, is an ancient type of complementary medicine and is one of the most trusted fields in the medical area. In several countries, Ayurveda is still considered a main part of the healthcare system. According to ayurvedic experts, this ancient type of medicinal field is based on the theory that the combination of space, earth, air, fire, and water makes up an individual. Together, these elements form energies or humors known as Doshas. There are three main doshas in ayurvedic medicine such as:

- Vata dosha

- Pitta dosha

- Kapha dosha

In terms of Ayurvedic medicine, all illnesses are due to fluctuation in the doshas of a person and ayurvedic experts will treat the illness by rebalancing these humors. In ayurvedic medicines, diet, exercise, meditation, herbal medicines, breathing exercises, and physical therapy are used along with several other methods. Whatever technique or method is used, the primary goal of all treatments is to restore the balance between body, mind, and spirit.

SHILAJIT AND AYURVEDIC MEDICINE

Shilajit is an important part of Ayurvedic medicine with a long history of being used as a tonic and a rejuvenating agent. It is a mineral-rich substance that is obtained when the hydrocarbon-rich material decomposes. This black, sticky resin is known to have a wide range of health benefits and can be used as a potent Ayurvedic medicine. Shilajit is a potent and effective Ayurvedic medicine that helps in correcting hormonal imbalances, strengthening the nervous system, improving digestion, boosting the immune system, and even aiding in weight loss. Shilajit improves the complexion, promotes hair growth, and prevents hair loss. It is also known to improve eyesight and is very helpful in treating headaches and other neurological disorders like epilepsy and Parkinson's disease.

No doubt, shilajit is a very popular ayurvedic remedy for treating many conditions and diseases. However, it is important to note that shilajit is a strong medicine and must be taken under supervision. The recommended dosage for shilajit is 2-3 grams (1 gm = 1000 mg) of the resin per day in powder form. The powder has a bitter taste and should be mixed with a little water or milk and taken twice a day, in the morning and evening. You can also take shilajit as a paste by mixing it with a little water or ghee and applying it on the forehead, the temples, or any other part of the body where the veins are visible.

HISTORY OF SHILAJIT USE

After the unusual discovery of shilajit by monkeys (as mentioned above in the section "Shilajit in Modern Times"), the natives became curious about the sudden health changes and improved wellness in the monkeys. Therefore, they started using the same blackish substance extracted from rocks and said that they felt more energetic, had better stamina, and observed improvement in overall health. After that, local practitioners also started to use shilajit in their practice and claimed that it provides relief from digestive problems, enhances sexual activity, improves cognitive skills, increases energy levels, improves memory, and many more. Due to these curative and healing approaches, traditional practitioners increased the use of shilajit and also formulated methods to purify it.

A brief insight into the history of shilajit is given in the following points:

- Shilajit is an important therapeutic substance that was used by Hindu physicians for the treatment of a number of diseases.

- According to a discipline of ayurvedic, The Caraka Samhita, the shilajit lays the foundation of the modern-day rejuvenating agent.

- According to Caraka Samhita, when shilajit is administered to a healthy person, it produces incredible levels of energy.

- In another approach of ayurvedic medicine, the Sushruta Samhita, when shilajit is taken slowly in adequate doses, it shows significant improvements in the physical strength of the body and enhances the skin complexion

- In the Astanga Hrdayam, the ancient discipline of ayurvedic, it is mentioned that the shilajit is the best rejuvenator.

USE OF SHILAJIT IN AYURVEDIC MEDICINE

From the records, it has been proved that shilajit was an integral part of the ayurvedic practice and still, it has been used by people all over the world. Shilajit has been used for following health concerns in ancient times and still now, people are using it for treating similar disorders.

1) For anemia

Anemia is a disorder that is caused by a decline in the number of red blood cells or a reduction in the levels of hemoglobin in the blood. Among all, iron deficiency anemia is the most prevalent type of anemia. Anemia is characterized by fatigue, general weakness, dizziness, pale skin, and many similar symptoms. People in the past noticed that by taking shilajit, they regained energy, their skin complexion returned to normal, and there was relief from the other symptoms of anemia such as dizziness, shortness of breath, and irregular heartbeats. Thus, our ancestors became greatly dependent on shilajit to treat life-threatening diseases including anemia. Even today, people often take shilajit as a dietary supplement to increase hemoglobin levels and to increase the count of red blood cells.

2) For Heart Health

In the past, shilajit was often taken to improve heart health and wellness because shilajit was found to cope with irregular heartbeats, alleviate chest pain, prevent shortness of breath, improve circulation, and induce energy. Various clinical studies have been done to find out whether this concept of shilajit is authentic or not, and as expected, shilajit provided beneficial effects on stabilizing lipid levels and enhancing overall heart health. Hence, relying on shilajit in ancient times was the right decision and is now even proven by the latest research.

3) For muscle fatigue

As mentioned before, monkeys showed more energy and agility after licking the black sticky material released by rocks so, people also took interest in that black substance and utilized it to gain similar advantages. Consequently, people felt more alive, and active, and were able to get rid of muscular pain and tiredness. Thus, in those days, shilajit became a natural healer to deal with fatigue and exhaustion, and due to this, people experienced high levels of energy. Even today, people are using shilajit supplements to get rid of fatigue caused by exercises or other strenuous physical activities and to boost muscular strength.

4) For Mental Health

Shilajit was found to reduce memory-related problems and people were taking it to improve their mental performance and combat mental issues. Previously, people were unaware of the fact why shilajit was so effective in mental health but in light of the latest research, it was found that shilajit contains fulvic acid and certain amino acids that can enhance memory and boost mental health. Even some studies claim that shilajit can reduce the risk of Alzheimer's disease which is a severe brain disorder and is also responsible for mental disability.

5) For Gastric ulcers

A gastric ulcer or peptic ulcer is a gastric disorder in which the lining of the stomach gets exposed to damaging agents or conditions such as free radicals and oxidative stress that could lead to severe stomach lesions. In old times, when people consume shilajit, they got relief from stomach pain and issues in their digestive tract. Plus, there was a significant improvement in digestion. This is due to the anti-inflammatory, and antioxidant activities of shilajit, and therefore, shilajit is considered a beneficial supplement for stomach ulcers.

6) For aging

Shilajit gained popularity for its rejuvenating properties and anti-aging effects. People were attracted to these blackish-brown mountain secretions because they helped them to retain their youthfulness. People experienced improved wellness and strength, felt more energetic, and thus, believed that shilajit had reversed the effects of aging. Thus, it would not be wrong to say, it was the antiaging benefits of shilajit that was the reason for its popularity and grasped everyone's attention.

A number of studies concluded that the anti-aging and rejuvenating benefits of shilajit are due to the presence of vital minerals, potent anti-inflammatory agents, antioxidants, and fulvic acid that protect the body from free radical damage and also slow down the natural phenomena of aging.

7) For other purposes

Shilajit was a favorite alternative of our ancestors for dealing with several common problems including:

- Lethargy

- Seasonal depression

- Physical weakness

- Sleeping disorders

- Edema

- Mountain sickness

- Appetite disorders

People reported positive outcomes after using shilajit for the above health issues and continued its use because of its amazing healing and curative benefits. Medical experts theorized that the medicinal profile of shilajit is largely due to the presence of fulvic acid, amino acids, and certain other essential minerals.

CONCLUSIONS

Ayurvedic medicine is a vital part of the ancient medical system and its foundation is based on ancient writings. These writings are according to the natural and holistic approaches that are tailored to the well-organized treatment of diseases and betterment of physical and mental health. In the ayurvedic approach to disease management, treatment is derived from the combination of plants, animals, metals, minerals, diet, exercise, and lifestyle. Among all, the use of shilajit is the prominent one. Shilajit has appeared in the therapeutic history of various cultures and is, therefore, known as a favorite healing agent of ancient times. Shilajit has been extensively used in ayurvedic medicine for centuries and still now, people are using this miraculous natural gift to improve their standard of living. This black substance carries the therapeutic powers of the mountains gifted by nature and is shaping the world of nutraceuticals due to its uncountable medicinal powers.

CHAPTER #3:
SHILAJIT AND THE LATEST DISCOVERIES

You have now become quite familiar with the origin, discovery, and composition of shilajit. Plus, an overview of effectiveness and benefits along with the detailed history of shilajit is also given in the previous chapters. It is interesting to know how people in the past were using shilajit to boost their energy levels and enhance their health. Our forefathers were totally dependent on natural healing methods including herbal remedies, ayurvedic medicine, and similar therapies to fight mild health concerns like fever, headaches, cold, and flu, to life-threatening, serious illnesses like heart issues, kidney disorders, and illnesses that occur due to the deficiencies of several essential minerals. Most of these therapeutic discoveries are still in practice and the global use of shilajit is one of them.

Shilajit offers many advantages and is emerging as a favorite dietary supplement. Although people are not that much familiar with the benefits of shilajit and often use other alternatives, now after extensive clinical trials and in light of contemporary research, people are becoming more aware of this natural healer and incorporating its use in their daily lives.

USES OF SHILAJIT: BACKED BY RESEARCHES

Shilajit has branches in various fields of the therapeutic world and one can notice the presence of shilajit in every culture since its discovery. From boosting sexual health, mental power, and physical strength to proving itself the best healing therapy for mild to severe pathologies, shilajit stands out as a unique endowment of nature. This is the reason why shilajit has become a favorite topic of discussion among health experts and why a lot of research work has been done to figure out more about shilajit. Although shilajit is beneficial in every aspect of medical and health sciences, its role is more promising in specific diseases and conditions.

Some of these disorders are briefly discussed below:

ALZHEIMER'S DISEASE

Alzheimer's disease is the most prevalent form of dementia that is a progressive brain disorder. It initiates with memory loss that is insignificant in its early stages but gradually, it worsens and results in the inability to perform daily life activities, for example, carrying on normal conversations with others becomes difficult, and normal responses to common external stimuli are also compromised. This is because Alzheimer's disease influences those parts of the brain that are involved in controlling thoughts, memories, and language. Alzheimer's disease is common among older people and its risk and severity increase with the age. The initial symptoms appear after the age of 60 and this disease is less common among young people. Some of the most common symptoms of Alzheimer's disease include:

- Memory impairment is the initial sign of the disease
- Abrupt changes in mood and personality

- Difficulty in doing and completing easy tasks at home or workplace

- Declining mental health and poor cognitive skills

- Difficulty in decision-making accompanied by poor judgment skills

- As the disease progresses, memory loss becomes more prominent and creates an alarming situation

Alzheimer's has now become a serious health concern and its prevalence is also increasing at a dangerously higher rate. Owing to the severity of the disease, experts are looking for treatment options that are most effective and easily available to everyone. Besides medical approaches and psychotherapy, a fast increase in the use of nutraceuticals or dietary supplements is also recorded. Among them, the herbal remedy of shilajit is the most noticeable. According to research published by the "International Journal of Ayurveda Research", it was found that shilajit can be used as an effective therapy for the treatment of Alzheimer's and Parkinson's diseases. According to this study, shilajit possesses immunostimulant, anti-inflammatory, and antioxidative strength that can reduce toxicity in the brain and reduce inflammation, and eventually, reverse the symptoms of the disease and also complement other treatments tailored towards the management of Alzheimer's disease.

Similarly, another study was conducted by the "Asian Journal of Research in Pharmaceutical Science" to find out the effectiveness of shilajit in the management of Alzheimer's disease. This clinical trial concluded that the shilajit, being rich in humic substances and fulvic acid, can reduce inflammation and can also prevent the abnormal build-up of proteins in the brain that are responsible for inducing the symptoms of Alzheimer's. Moreover, shilajit is also found to block the signals that may trigger Alzheimer's and reinforce the effects of other targeted therapies.

FERTILITY

Shilajit is also known to improve fertility in both men and women. From the very beginning, people of Indian territory were using shilajit to treat the issues with their reproductive system and fertility. In modern times, the use of shilajit is still in practice and many ayurvedic practitioners widely recommend the use of shilajit to treat fertility issues.

Due to higher rates of successful cases, medical researchers also working on the shilajit to know whether it really helps with fertility or if it is just a myth! Unexpectedly, shilajit provides positive outcomes and is found to greatly enhance the reproductive health and fertility of both males and females.

Take an example of a study called "Clinical Evaluation of Spermatogenic Activity of Processed Shilajit in Oligospermia" that examined the effects of shilajit in 60 infertile patients. These patients were given shilajit in, the form of a capsule, after every meal, two times a day, and for 90 days. After 90 days, all participants were asked to provide their semen samples. On examining the semen of each participant, it was found that 61% of men had an increase in total sperm count, 37% have shown improvements in sperm production while 12-17% showed an increase in sperm motility (the ability of sperm to move efficiently).

In another study published in the "Journal of Ethnopharmacology", the ability of shilajit to produce sperm in males and stimulate the release of eggs in females is studied thoroughly. According to this, there was a significant increase in sperm count and an increase in the size of male reproductive organs while in females, there was an early release of an egg. Moreover, in females, shilajit is also found to increase the supply of oxygen to reproductive organs, help in having a normal menstrual cycle, reduce excess body fat, and eventually prepare the female body to conceive.

IRON DEFICIENCY ANEMIA

Iron deficiency anemia is the most common type of anemia that occurs due to a deficiency of red blood cells or hemoglobin in the blood. Hemoglobin is a protein, present in red blood cells, that is required to carry oxygen throughout the body including all vital organs and tissues of the body. Due to low levels of iron in the blood, red blood cells failed to produce enough amount of hemoglobin and as a result, the quality of red blood also decreases resulting in the blood disorder called anemia. Anemia presents with the following symptoms:

- Unexplained fatigue and tiredness

- Pale, yellowish skin

- Brittle nails

- Headaches

- Dizziness

- Shortness of breath and chest pain

- General weakness

- Urges to eat unusual things such as paper, ice, dirt, etc

- A significant decrease in appetite

Iron deficiency anemia is usually asymptomatic in its initial stages and therefore, left unnoticed. But as time passes, anemia becomes severe and requires extensive treatments, otherwise, it could become fatal.

In the majority of cases, iron deficiency anemia can be corrected by supplements. Doctors often recommend Vitamin C and iron supplements but these supplements are heavy and could cause side effects like stomach issues, change in the color of urine and stools, nausea, tooth staining, stomach cramps, etc. Therefore, people often look for natural remedies including herbal supplements such as shilajit. Being enriched with humic acid and iron content, shilajit become a popular dietary supplement to cope with iron deficiencies. The effectiveness of shilajit is further confirmed by a study published by the "Asian Pacific Journal of Tropical Biomedicine" that evaluates the usefulness of shilajit. This study proposed that shilajit can be used as a dietary supplement, without any side effects, for several disorders including iron deficiency anemia. Another study, known as "Shilajit in management of iron deficiency anemia" provided similar conclusions. According to this, regular, controlled doses of shilajit can increase the level of hemoglobin and the number of healthy red blood cells in anemic patients and proves that shilajit has strong anti-anemic powers.

ANTIAGING

Shilajit is the oldest known remedy for staying younger and retaining youth. Shilajit performs its anti-aging duty by slowing down the natural process of aging. Cell damage and free radicals are one of the biggest culprits behind aging. The antioxidant and anti-inflammatory agents, that are present in abundance in the shilajit, target those free radicals and other cell-damaging factors and destroy them. Moreover, these antioxidant and anti-inflammatory properties, together with fulvic acid, repair cell damage, prevent deterioration of the body caused by aging, removes wrinkles and fine lines, boost energy levels, and prevent the external manifestations as well as internal effects of aging.

Shilajit has been known for its rejuvenating abilities since its discovery and still, people all over the world are using it to rejuvenate themselves and restore their youth. A review named "Shilajit: A Medicinal Mystery to Cure the Un-cure Disease" thoroughly explores various clinical trials that point out the antiaging and rejuvenating activities of shilajit. This review found that the majority of studies were in favor of shilajit and they emphasized the use of shilajit to reverse the effects of aging and to rejuvenate oneself.

Another research "Chemistry of Shilajit, An immunomodulatory Ayurvedic Rasayan" theorized that the antiaging benefits of shilajit are due to immunomodulatory agents and the ability of shilajit to influence the hormonal system of the body. In short, the presence of essential minerals, amino acids, and important metals increases the worth of shilajit and it stands out as a most effective antiaging supplement.

DIABETES

Diabetes has now become a leading health concern with every 1 out of 10 people being the victim of it and according to reports, about 10% of the total world population has been diagnosed with diabetes. If appropriate actions are not taken on time, then the prevalence of diabetes is expected to increase at alarming rates in the near future. Diabetes is caused by the high level of glucose in the blood that is regulated by the hormone insulin under normal circumstances. Sometimes, the body is not able to utilize insulin or there might be a deficiency of insulin due to any reasons. This will, in turn, lead to a metabolic disorder, known as diabetes, which is characterized by dangerously high levels of blood glucose. The early signs and symptoms of diabetes are:

- Frequent urges to urinate especially at night

- Unexplained weight loss

- Early exhaustion or extreme tiredness

- Increase appetite

- Feeling thirsty all time

- Dry mouth

- Wounds that heal slowly

- Vision problems

- Increase complaints of infections

- Numbing or tingling sensation in hands and feet

Diabetes is a chronic and life-threatening illness but by early diagnosis, one can properly manage it and minimize its fatality. By balanced diet, exercises, stress management, and taking prescribe medications according to schedule, you can not only live a normal life but can also reverse its symptoms. Along with these, doctors often recommend supplements that not only protect from the dangers of the disease but also improve the efficacy of the medical therapies. For supplements, the use of shilajit is the most promising one, and doctors usually advise opting for natural therapies instead of chemically synthesized supplements.

The antidiabetic role of diabetes is further explored by several experimental studies that provide results in the favor of shilajit. For example, a study in the "Indian Journal of Pharmacology" examined whether the administration of shilajit in diabetic subjects can reduce the levels of glucose and lipid in the serum. As expected from the experiment, there was a significant reduction in the blood glucose levels confirming the glucose-lowering ability of shilajit. Besides, a review published by "Phytotherapy Research" concluded that the antidiabetic benefits of shilajit are due to the presence of fulvic acid that reduces the oxidative stress in the body and provide protection against inflammation, thus, preventing the risk of type 2 diabetes and can also help in its management. Similarly, another review given in the "Journal of Ethnopharmacology" go through the traditional use of shilajit in Indian medicine. According to this review, shilajit is often used along with milk to control diabetes and the ongoing practice of this method proved that shilajit is extremely beneficial for diabetic patients and therefore, should be used in controlled doses and after the expert's opinion.

CANCER

Just like diabetes, cancer is another serious disorder that is feared all over the world and is characterized by abnormal and uncontrolled cell growth. It is an even more serious and deteriorating disease than diabetes and other chronic, life-threatening illnesses. Cancer now emerges as the second leading cause of death and its prevalence is increasing at a very threatening rate. But luckily, with the advancement in medical science, the survival rate of cancer has been improving. The signs and symptoms of cancer are not apparent in its initial stages and sometimes, people even didn't know they have cancer until they become seriously ill or develop pain that becomes unbearable. Further, the symptoms of cancer are general and it is difficult to predict cancer merely according to such symptoms. For proper confirmation, there is a need for medical tests and diagnosis. Anyhow, some of the symptoms that can be seen in every type of cancer are:

- Idiopathic body pain that is constant
- Formation of lump or mass that are palpable
- Indigestion
- Extreme fatigue and laziness
- Anemia and bleeding without any reason
- Prominent weight loss or gain
- Poor wound healing

- The difficulty is breathing and swallowing

- Changes in skin color and bruising

- Fever that is untreatable

Although it is difficult to avoid cancer if you are at risk, however, by lifestyle modification and early diagnosis, you can live a healthy, cancer-free life. For the treatment, there are several options available. Some types of treatment will target the specific type of cancer and the affected body area such as radiation therapy while other treatments will provide a systematic approach including medications and supplements. Cancer is an extremely serious condition that needs proper and specialized medical attention but according to certain studies, some dietary supplements particularly shilajit can do wonders for cancer prevention and management if taken properly and according to required doses.

There is extensive research work on the benefits of shilajit and the majority of them proved that shilajit is beneficial when it comes to cancer. For instance, a study given in the *"International Journal of Toxicological and Pharmacological Research"* reviewed the anti-cancer ability of shilajit. According to this, shilajit comprises humic acid and fulvic acid which are known for their potent anti-inflammatory, antioxidant, antitumor, and antitoxic properties. That's why shilajit can be used in cancer therapy as a chemotherapeutic agent and also in the prevention of cancer. Moreover, shilajit can kill cancerous cells without causing any harm to normal cells, unlike other chemotherapies. In another research given in *"Scientific reports"* that was done on the cancerous cells of the urinary bladder, it was observed that the mumio (shilajit) performed selective action and killed the cancerous cells while the normal cells remain intact. This study proved that shilajit also has apoptotic properties in which it performs targeted functions by killing unwanted, harmful cells and doesn't harm normal cells. Besides, shilajit not only proves itself a promising natural medicine for cancer management and prevention but it can also protect and treat the damage caused by chemotherapy. In a clinical study published in *"Archives of Gynecology and Obstetrics"*, it was shown that the radiation therapy used for the treatment of ovarian cancer can lead to noticeable cellular and chromosomal damage. This radiation-induced damage is treatable and preventable by taking controlled doses of shilajit for a specific time period.

MENTAL HEALTH

Your brain and body are the main pillars of life. A balance between them is necessary if you want to live a life full of peace and wellness. But unfortunately, most of us lost this balance and consequently, our lives get out of our hands. People often keep a strict check on their physical selves and forget about their mental health. This is the reason why there is an alarming increase in the ratio of mental disorders with depression, anxiety, and stress at the top of the list. Moreover, the rate of suicide is also increasing.

To cope with such situations and to achieve genuine prosperity in life, a healthy mind is very important and even more important than physical health. And here, shilajit comes as an ultimate savior. Shilajit is equally useful for your mental well-being as it is for your body. In the past, when there was no existence of psychotherapy and other particular treatments for the mind, people were using herbs and other natural drugs to enhance their psychological and emotional state. The use of shilajit was one of them. Even today, shilajit is in high demand because of its ability to boost mood, relieve stress and anxiety, improve sleep quality, and to confirm this, a bunch of medical studies have been done on the effects of shilajit on mental health. A study named *"Energy and Health Benefits of Shilajit"*, demonstrated the physical and mental benefits of shilajit on the human body. The study states that, due to the presence of potent minerals and acids, the shilajit acts as a revitalizer and promotes mental health by reducing mental fatigue and promoting other neurogenic effects. In another study, the antidepressant properties of shilajit were studied. This study was published in the *"Asian Journal of Pharmacology & Toxicology"* and it concluded that unlike other pharmaceutical therapies for depression that cause severe side effects, shilajit produced prominent antidepressive effects without causing any side effects. Besides direct beneficial effects on the mind, studies reveal that shilajit is also indirectly involved in the protection of mental health and in the prevention of neurodegenerative diseases too.

Coenzyme Q10 is a natural antioxidant produced by the body that is responsible for the growth and maintenance of cells and provides protection against neurodegenerative brain diseases and mental disorders. Shilajit is found to rejuvenate Coenzyme Q10 and enhance its functioning and thus, contribute towards the prevention of mental disorders.

CONCLUSIONS

No wonder, why our ancestors were a fan of this natural medicine and why its use is still so popular even after the discovery of thousands of conventional treatment methods. A large number of reviews, research, clinical trials, and medical experiments further prove the miraculous nature of shilajit. Shilajit can be used for numerous other health conditions too that include both physical and mental health. For example, many pieces of research support the effectiveness of shilajit in enhancing sleep quality, its antiseptic properties, diuretic effects, and immunity-boosting strength. But the clinical trials on these subjects is limited and most of the experiment are done on animals. Therefore, there is a need for more experimental studies on humans to further confirm these therapeutic effects of Shilajit.

However, the best part of using shilajit is that it comes with no potential side effects and it performs targeted functions making it even more favorable and preferable. But one thing you should keep in mind is to never replace prescribed medications or therapies with natural remedies and if you are planning to use any natural treatment, it would be best to consult a field expert first. In this way, you can protect yourself from any side effects, and eventually, you will be able to extract maximum benefits from natural remedies including   Shilajit.

CHAPTER #4
GENERAL HEALTH BENEFITS OF SHILAJIT

Shilajit is often referred to as the "Destroyer of Weakness" in Ayurvedic medicine due to its unbeatable quality of rejuvenation. For centuries, shilajit has been used as the most reliable healer for all sorts of problems related to health. As, shilajit is a product of decomposition exclusively secreted by the mountains, natives of nearby regions are getting more benefits from this natural remedy. The presence of biologically active molecules, minerals, metals, and other potent trace elements make shilajit a much-needed antidote for better physical and mental health. Shilajit derived its main powers from the fulvic acid and that's why it has remained a crucial element in curative medicine. It would not be wrong to say that shilajit is the precursor of the nutraceutical world due to its energy-boosting, anti-inflammatory, memory, cognitive skill-enhancing, immunomodulatory, antiaging, antioxidant, antitoxic, and antidiuretic properties. Besides, shilajit is also found to possess strong adaptogenic, antitumor, antibacterial, antiviral, anti-anemic, and antidiabetic powers that double its therapeutic values.

In short, the healing benefits of shilajit are beyond the scope of a single book and it is not possible to cover them in a single spot. Still, through this chapter, you will get to know some of the well-known curative skills of shilajit and how this natural healer is shaping the health and medical world because of its exceptional medicinal powers.

MENTAL BENEFITS

Shilajit is a natural herb that is gifted with uncountable nutrients, vitamins, and other essential minerals. All these active contents of shilajit are believed to have innumerable benefits for mental health that can overcome anxiety attacks, prevent anxiety disorder, reduce stress, and treat depression. With this, shilajit can stimulate the production of dopamine in the brain and therefore, is beneficial for inducing mental peace and pleasure. Although there is a need for specialized medical treatments and therapies for serious mental disorders like depression, anxiety, etc., the application of shilajit as a supplement can be used as a catalyst for other therapies and may also help in preventing serious mental problems at first place, as proven by medical studies.

The in-depth details of shilajit's role in mental health are given below:

- **Cognitive development**

Cognitive development is based on the ability of a person to think, remember, learn, and concentrate. Shilajit is a neuroprotective nutraceutical enriched with fulvic acid and vital antioxidants that provokes cognitive development and enhance cognitive skills. It also put a pause on brain aging. Regular consumption of shilajit can improve focus, concentration, alertness, memory, decision-making, and learning skills, and significantly reduce the risk of disorders that may lead to declining mental performance and cognitive skills.

- **Reduce stress**

Shilajit is best known as a stress killer. Stress is something that arises due to external triggers and it worsens due to poor mental control. Moreover, stress can also have a huge impact on physical and mental health and a majority of physical and psychological illnesses could become worse due to uncontrolled stress. As indicated by a study, shilajit can reduce stress due to the presence of amino acids particularly "tyrosine" and also by inhibiting the production of stress hormones called, cortisol, and adrenaline. Thus, shilajit can be used as a stress healer without a second thought.

- **Mood enhancer**

To uplift mood, shilajit can be used as a magic pill that will not only function as an anti-stressor but can also combat your mood swings effectively. Shilajit uses the same mechanisms to enhance the mood that helps in the alleviation of stress.

- **Antidepressant effect**

For depression, there are many treatments and methods that can provide successful outcomes but they might provide superficial, short-term relief and are also expected to cause potential side effects. Thus, experts are always looking for natural ways that are reliable with long-term benefits and side effects. Shilajit perfectly fulfills this criterion and so, is regarded as a most competent natural remedy. The deficiency of zinc is one of the major reasons behind depression and shilajit contains zinc as one of its vital minerals. The regular intake of shilajit can fulfill zinc requirements and thus, can be used as a natural antidepressant. Besides, other mineral content of shilajit including amino acids and fulvic acid is also useful in the treatment of depression. Also, a study showed that shilajit can increase the levels of neurotransmitters in the brain, known as Gamma-aminobutyric acid (GABA). GABA functions as a soothing chemical that reduces stress and anxiety, induces mental relaxation and minimizes the signs and symptoms of depression.

- **Enhance memory skills**

Shilajit promotes mental health and improves memory due to its magical natural contents. A trace element, dibenzo-alpha-pyrone, present in shilajit is very important in boosting memory and thinking skills. This trace element prevents the breakdown of essential chemicals in the brain that is needed for good memory and can also delay mental aging.

- **Shilajit doses for Mental health**

The recommended dose of shilajit is 250-1000 mg which can be taken with milk or water. Doctors advise taking two doses per day, one, in the morning on an empty stomach and the other before going to sleep.

TESTOSTERONE BOOSTERS

Testosterone is a male sex hormone that is essentially important for male sexual development. Its production decreases with age but sometimes, there is an abnormal decline in testosterone levels due to many reasons. The symptoms of low levels of the hormone are:

- Low sex drive is the primary symptoms

- Sexual dysfunction

- Depression, mood swings

- Unexplained fatigue

- Hair loss

- Increase in body fat and decrease in muscle mass

To combat testosterone deficiency, testosterone boosters are used worldwide. These boosters stimulate the production of testosterone and normalize its level in the body. The use of testosterone boosters was initially popular among athletes but now, the general population is also using them to fulfill their hormonal requirements. Now, medical studies also support the use of boosters and proposed that certain natural remedies can be as effective in promoting testosterone production as pharmaceutical interventions. For example, a clinical study was conducted on male adults who were under the age of 55 years. They were administrated with controlled doses of natural supplements including shilajit and after some time, the levels of testosterone were recorded. According to the results, there was a significant improvement in testosterone levels of more than half participants proving that shilajit can be used as an effective and safer testosterone booster. Another study provided similar results. In this study, young males were divided into two groups. One group was given placebo medicine and the other group was given 250 mg shilajit 2 times a day for 90 days. After 90 days, both groups were examined and according to the results, the group that was given shilajit had a significant increase in their testosterone levels.

IMPROVE SEXUAL ACTIVITY

It would not be wrong to say that shilajit is an all-in-one natural package. Among all the healing, therapeutic, and boosting skills of shilajit, the aphrodisiac property is the most significant. Aphrodisiac is the ability of a substance to induce sexual desire, pleasure, and attraction in both men and women. There is a huge industrial preparation of aphrodisiac drugs and supplements to improve sexual life. Besides, many natural alternatives are also known to possess aphrodisiac strengths including certain foods, aromatic oils, seeds, spices, and herbs.

Among all, shilajit is known as the strongest aphrodisiac agent from the time of its discovery and is still in use to increase libido, improve sexual health, and promote a better sexual life. The ways shilajit influences sexual performance are given below:

- **Increases libido**

Shilajit can boost libido and improve sexual performance, especially in men. This is due to the direct stimulation of male sex hormones that increases sexual desire and also enhances stamina during sexual activity.

- **Increase organ size**

Several studies also concluded that regular intake of shilajit can increase the size of male sex organs followed by the increased production of semen.

- **Treat impotency**

A research report claimed that shilajit can help in the treatment of impotency and premature ejaculation. Shilajit can combat erectile dysfunction due to its ability to increase blood flow to the sex organs and by managing other reasons for impotency including nutritional deficiencies, stress, weakness, and fatigue.

- **Increase sperm count**

Shilajit accelerates the production of sperm and that's why it is also known as a spermatogenic herb. A study showed that shilajit can increase sperm count by approximately 60 percent.

- **Enhance sexual performance**

Shilajit is also beneficial in enhancing sexual performance. It helps to maintain erection, reduces stress and anxiety that may suppress sexual arousal, prevents premature ejaculation due to the presence of antioxidants and minerals, and increases the blood flow to the sex organs.

- **Improves sperm motility**

In addition to increasing sperm count, shilajit can also improve sperm motility. Sperm motility is the movement of sperm and their ability to reach an egg. Good sperm motility is an indicator of male fertility and is necessary for reproduction. Shilajit can increase sperm motility by 50% and thus, can be used as a good dietary supplement to enhance male fertility.

- **Balance the hormonal level**

Shilajit helps to normalize the levels of female hormones including progesterone and estrogen. These are female reproductive hormones that promote good sexual performance in women by building stamina and improving libido.

- **Subside period irregularities**

By maintaining the normal levels of female sex hormones, shilajit supplements also treat period irregularities and ensure the normal duration and length of the monthly cycle. Moreover, shilajit is also used to alleviate period pain and cramps.

- **Stimulates ovulation**

Several studies and experts suggest that daily intake of shilajit can stimulate ovogenic effects in females. This means that shilajit can help in the treatment of female infertility and can stimulate the release of the egg by inducing ovulation.

APPLICATION OF SHILAJIT TO ENHANCE SPORTS PERFORMANCE

After extensive clinical trials and medical studies, shilajit has proven its therapeutic and curative properties. It is known as the best dietary supplement for improving health and lifestyle and also as a complementary therapy for serious disorders including cancer, diabetes, hypertension, blood disorders, Alzheimer's, and the list goes on. That's why experts suggest adding shilajit to your daily diet as a dietary supplement.

Besides being a promising natural healer, shilajit use is also noticeable when it comes to sports or workouts. The application of shilajit for enhancing sports performance is thoroughly explored and due to the significant influences of shilajit on athlete performance, its usage is becoming very popular.

Because of the following reasons, shilajit is extensively used for sports nutrition.

- **Energy booster**

According to studies, it was found that shilajit can increase the levels of ATP in the body by 10%. ATP is an organic molecule and is the main source of energy present in the body. For athletes or people who require a continuous supply of energy, shilajit would be the best option because it will not only provides energy but is also free from adverse side effects that are often seen with energy-boosting supplements.

- **Improve stamina**

Besides an energy booster, shilajit is also used for boosting stamina. Usually, sports are high-impact activities that are intense and require continuous involvement. Due to this, individuals often become exhausted and lost their stamina. But, using shilajit during training sessions or before a particular event, you can naturally increase your stamina and make it possible to go through tough situations without getting tired.

- **Physical performance**

By boosting stamina and energy, shilajit automatically ensures better physical performance. In addition to this, taking shilajit is also linked with an improved supply of oxygen and blood to organs and tissues including muscles and the nervous system. Due to an increase in blood and nutrient circulation to the brain and muscles, physical performance becomes better, and the chances of winning doubles.

- **Better cardiovascular strength**

Shilajit is also found to increase cardiovascular strength and performance. A study found that consuming controlled doses of shilajit promotes a better supply of oxygen, blood, and other nutrients to the heart, thus, improving endurance and blood circulation during sports. It has also been observed that those athletes who have taken shilajit have stable serum levels of cholesterol and lipids.

- **Vasodilates blood vessels**

One of the significant discoveries about shilajit is its ability to dilate blood vessels and promotes blood supply to muscles during strenuous physical activities. The research concluded that shilajit can increase the amounts of nitric oxide (NO) in the body which is known for its role in dilating the blood vessels. NO causes an increase in blood and nutrients flow to the cells, especially to the muscle cells. Thus, those individuals who take shilajit during training sessions or before participating in any sports, show better performance, endurance, and stamina as compared to others.

- **Prevent iron deficiency**

Iron deficiency is often observed in those who have to go through vigorous training sessions, especially in women, because of monthly blood loss due to menstruation. Therefore, shilajit, being packed with iron content, can help you to combat iron loss effectively.

- **Strengthen muscles**

Shilajit strengthens the skeletal muscles by promoting the synthesis of collagen production. In research, it was found that shilajit consumption increases the strength, flexibility, and endurance of skeletal muscles by causing an increase in the production of collagen and proteins and also helps to repair and regenerate muscle cells.

- **Improves mental health**

For athletes, it is necessary to have mental peace and relaxation, otherwise, their performance will be not according to expectations. Here, shilajit again saves the day and ensures a better mental state. Shilajit can improve focus, cognitive skills, memory, reduce stress, tension, anxiety, and mental fatigue, and clear your mind so that you can focus on your performance.

- **Best for recovery**

During sports or other physical activities, injuries are very common and they might reduce your performance and even threaten your participation. The use of shilajit as a dietary supplement promotes your sports performance and also promotes quick recovery. It is stuffed with anti-inflammatories and antioxidants and because of this, wounds, cuts, bruises, or other sports injuries are easy to heal with regular use of shilajit.

SHILAJIT FOR WORKOUTS

The use of shilajit is extremely beneficial for those who regularly workouts such as fitness freaks, health enthusiasts, and bodybuilders, or those who are doing any sort of exercise. During the workout, muscles undergo minor tears followed by high levels of muscular stress and injuries. In the absence of proper rest and healthy nutrition, muscles may take longer than usual to heal and may eventually lead to muscular pain and general weakness. To avoid such conditions, shilajit can be used as an ideal supplement to boost muscle strength and promote effective and quick healing. Shilajit is often consumed as a pre-workout supplement.

Pre-workout Supplement

Pre-work supplements are dietary supplements that are taken prior to a workout or exercise. These pre-workout supplements act as fuel for your body that will help you to keep going without getting tired because such supplements are intended to provide you with the required nutrients and minerals. Shilajit is recognized as one of these pre-workout supplements that provide you with a boost of energy needed for the workout. It also helps in maintaining the glucose levels in the blood during the activity. You can get hundreds of minerals, metals, essential organic molecules, and other nutrients from a single dose of shilajit. In a nutshell, shilajit can help you in the following ways:

- Fulvic acid is rich in oxygen content which helps in boosting endurance and prevent muscle soreness, shortness of breath, and fatigue caused by continuous physical activity

- The mineral and metal composition of shilajit will provide you with enough muscular strength during the workout

- Shilajit is an energy booster that fuels your body and helps in restoring energy throughout the activity by converting carbohydrates into energy.

- Being rich in electrolytes, shilajit maintains the water balance in the body. Moreover, shilajit can also help you to stay hydrated. The recommended dose for pre-workout shilajit intake is 300 to 500 mg per day.

CHAPTER #5
HOW SHILAJIT WORKS?

Shilajit was one of the oldest remedies known to mankind. People were using it even though there were no strong shreds of evidence supporting the use of shilajit. They observed the promising effects of blackish tar-like material on animals and their curiosity forced them to experience it on themselves even though they didn't know its constituents and were unfamiliar with the mechanism of action behind it. Even there was the frequent use of raw shilajit obtained directly from the mountains which were stuffed with huge amounts of impurities. Despite all, there was no reduction in its usage and its popularity is still blooming while providing never-ending medicinal benefits. As time passed and with the latest developments in the health industry, experts turned their attention toward the shilajit and started to work on extracting the purest and high-quality shilajit. They also tried to figure out the exact mechanism behind the shilajit action and strength to treat a number of diseases. Moreover, experts started exploring the various aspects of ayurvedic medicine and initiate their research on the active ingredients of ayurvedic therapies including shilajit. All these efforts lead to several remarkable discoveries that pointed out the exact process according to which shilajit works and also elaborated the active components of shilajit that define its healing and curative profiles.

ACTIVE INGREDIENTS OF SHILAJIT

The amazing power of shilajit is due to the presence of highly potent natural components that are known as active ingredients. An active ingredient is something that is biologically active and possesses healing properties. The main focus of active ingredients is to help in the diagnosis, treatment, and prevention of diseases by modulating the respective structure and function of the body. In the case of shilajit, the main active ingredients are humic acid and fulvic acid.

The shilajit consists of 60-80% of organic content, 20-40% mineral matter, and there is a presence of 5% of trace elements.

1) Organic Matter (60-80%)

It is the organic content of the shilajit that provides the major portion of medicinal benefits and comprises around 80% of all supplementary properties of shilajit. The organic portion of shilajit is produced by the decomposition of plants by microorganisms that combine with the remaining decomposed inorganic, mineral content, and trace elements. The organic content consists of humin, humic acid, and fulvic acids.

- **Humin**: It is an organic molecule that is insoluble in water at any pH and is naturally present in the soil. Humin enhances the physical and chemical properties of soil while, being the main part of shilajit, it is also beneficial for human health. Humin is an antioxidative substance and can be used to reduce oxidative stress in the body and for the treatment of ulcers.

- **Humic Acid**: Humic acid is an organic molecule that is water soluble under alkaline conditions. Basically, it is a chemical that is produced by decaying plants and helps the plant in getting water and nutrients. In herbal medicine, humic acid is considered an important therapeutic substance due to its beneficial medicinal effects on the immune system.

- **Fulvic Acid**: Among all organic chemicals, fulvic acid is the most useful one. It is soluble in water under various pH conditions and has low molecular weight. Fulvic acid has higher absorption rates in the intestine and can be excreted from the body within a few hours. Because of this, it is believed that the main portion of shilajit's medicinal properties is due to the fulvic acid, and therefore, during the extraction and purification of shilajit, major attention is given to its fulvic acid content.

It is important to know about the solubilities of organic content in water at different pH conditions because all the organic molecules operate according to their solubilities in water and, the fulvic acid, being more water soluble, is considered the most effective one. Other organic molecules of shilajit include phenolic acid, polyphenols, sterols, amino acids, 3,4-benzocoumarins, triterpenes, polysaccharides, lignins, resins, eldagic acids, latex, albumins, gums, and aromatic carboxylic acids.

2) Mineral matter (20-40%)

Minerals are known as the inorganic composition of shilajit and they are required for ensuring the nutritional benefits of the shilajit. There are approximately 84 or more active minerals present in the shilajit that act as an energy booster, perform antioxidative and anti-inflammatory functions, stabilize the level of blood cells, improve memory, and enhance overall health. Some of the important minerals found in shilajit include selenium, iron, calcium, copper, silica, antimony, lithium, molybdenum, manganese, zinc, sodium, and phosphorus.

3) Trace elements (5%)

There are some trace elements too in the shilajit that perform their own characteristic functions. For example, a trace element called, dibenzo-α-pyrones, acts as a carrier of other substances and also works together with fulvic acid to carry out major functions of shilajit.

MECHANISM OF ACTION

The mechanism of action is based on the quality of shilajit and the number of bioactive ingredients present in it. Shilajit is produced by the prolonged decomposition of plants, animals, and other minerals between the layers of the mountain. After a considerable time when the temperature of surrounding regions becomes high, shilajit is released from the mountains in its raw form. In unpurified form, shilajit is of black color that is sticky and gooey material. After purification, shilajit becomes free from impurities and is ready for use. Shilajit is purified and can be used for various health conditions. The way shilajit acts and provides medicinal effects is totally dependent upon the condition to be treated. As a whole, shilajit is known for its curative benefits because of the presence of the following properties that define the ability of shilajit to work in the body:

- **Antioxidant**

  An antioxidant mode of action is one in which chemicals or antioxidants will prevent or reduce the cellular and tissue damage caused by free radicals. Free radicals are unstable atoms that are produced during cell metabolism and could lead to severe damage to cells.

- **Anti-inflammatory**

Anti-inflammatory mechanisms in shilajit boost immunity, reduce oxidative stress, and prevent the accumulation of toxins that may contribute to inflammation.

- **Antidiuretics**

Shilajit helps to balance the level of water, salt, and other fluids in the body and thus, acts as a natural antidiuretic.

- **Antiseptic**

The antiseptic action of shilajit is due to the presence of particular acids such as benzoic acid which acts antibacterial and humic acid which acts as an antiviral.

- **Antidiabetic**

Shilajit's antidiabetic mode of action is due to the presence of antioxidants and fulvic acid that stabilizes blood glucose levels.

- **Cholinomimetic effects**

Cholinomimetic effects produced by shilajit mimic the action of a natural chemical produced in the brain (acetylcholine) that is responsible for controlling attention, memory, and learning skills.

- **Antianemia**

Iron is one of the major mineral contents of the shilajit. Therefore, shilajit can be used as an effective dietary supplement to cope with iron deficiency disorders including anemia.

- **Adaptogenic**

Adaptogenic agents refer to herbs or other substances that help the body to accommodate the fluctuating physical and emotional stresses that often occur in the residents of high altitudes. From the beginning, shilajit has been in use to combat health problems caused by living at high altitudes such as insomnia, motion sickness, hypoxia, breathing disorders, edema, and many others.

- **Antiaging**

The antiaging properties of shilajit are due to the presence of antioxidants and anti-inflammatory minerals. Moreover, shilajit is also involved in the production of collagen which is the major protein responsible for skin health and youthfulness.

- **Antidyslipidemic**

  The antidyslipidemic aspect of shilajit helps to stabilize the lipid profile by balancing the hormonal system of the body and controlling the serum cholesterol levels.

- **Antiepileptic**

  Shilajit controls seizures and epileptic attacks due to its strong antiepileptic properties. This mode of action, along with antipsychotics, also helps in the prevention of neurodegenerative disorders of the brain.

- **Anti-obesity**

  Shilajit has huge deposits of active components that can help the body to lose weight faster and get rid of excessive fats. Moreover, shilajit can suppress the appetite and prevents overeating. Thus, shilajit plays a vital role in the management of obesity and the reduction of weight in a shorter time period.

- **Spermatogenic**

Spermatogenic action is due to the ability of shilajit to influence the hormonal secretions and increase the levels of the testosterone hormone.

- **Ovogenic**

Ovogenic property of shilajit is due to its role in the regulation and stimulation of female sex hormones and in inducing the release of eggs.

- **Cardioprotective**

The cardioprotective mechanism is simply because of the abundance of antioxidants, anti-inflammatory, and rejuvenating agents in the shilajit.

- **Anticancer**

Anticancer effects of shilajit are caused by the selective killing of cancerous cells and causing no harm to normal cells. Moreover, shilajit's mechanism of action is largely based on its antitumor and antitoxic profiles.

SHILAJIT AND DISEASES

The medicinal benefits of shilajit are specific and its mode of action is strictly targeted to the condition for which it is used. A brief insight into the main points highlighting the process behind the shilajit and the condition it treats is given below:

- **Aging**

  The anti-aging and rejuvenating action of shilajit is due to the production of collagen, and the growth of new blood vessels and cells that protects the skin from the adverse effects of aging and improve skin microperfusion.

- **Energizer**

  Shilajit is rich in nutrients that the body needs. For example, being packed with iron, calcium, resin, zinc, magnesium, and similar minerals, shilajit can prevent fatigue and provide you with a long-term burst of energy.

- **Diabetes**

Shilajit shows potent antidiabetic effects due to the presence of antioxidants especially fulvic acid which regulates blood glucose levels and is also found to reduce the risk of diabetes.

- **Obesity**

The role of shilajit in reducing weight and shedding extra calories is the most noticeable. It has been used to control obesity and there are many successful cases of weight loss. Shilajit stimulates the rate of fat metabolism and suppresses hunger, and in this way, it helps to get rid of extra pounds.

- **Cancer**

The selective termination of tumor cells and apoptotic characteristics of shilajit make it a favorable addition to cancer therapy. Also, shilajit uses its antioxidant powers to repair the tissue damage caused by radiation therapy.

- **Alzheimer's disease**

The role of shilajit in Alzheimer's disease is extensively explained in previous sections. In short, shilajit can prevent the abnormal build-up of proteins in the brain that is responsible for causing Alzheimer's.

- **Heart health**

Due to its antioxidant, anti-inflammatory, energizing, and anti-toxic profile, shilajit is the best cardioprotective supplement that protects the heart from diseases and also enhances its functioning and strengthening.

- **Sexual health and performance**

Shilajit has been found to increase the size of male sex organs, stimulate the formation of sperm, and cause the production of the testosterone hormone. While for females, it can treat period irregularities and stimulate ovulation.

- **Stomach problems**

Shilajit can improve digestion and is also known as a gastroprotective agent that is an excellent remedy for the treatment of stomach ulcers. Shilajit can stimulate the synthesis of antioxidant enzymes that correct stomach lesions and repair damage caused by microbes, free radicals, or medicines.

- **Mental wellness**

Shilajit is found to improve mental health and uplift mood. This is because shilajit has the ability to stimulate the production of dopamine in the brain. This will, in turn, reduce anxiety, control stress, provide motivation, and boost mood. Besides, shilajit is also used as an antidepressant as it can increase the levels of serotonin hormone.

- **Antidiuretics**

There are also reports of the antidiuretic effects of shilajit. Antidiuretics balance fluid levels in the body and help the kidney to control the amount of water and salt in the body.

CONCLUSIONS

There is no specific mechanism that could explain the exact techniques behind the shilajit action. Instead, it is supposed that shilajit performs targeted actions and treats the condition for which it is taken while causing no effect on other body systems. This is the reason, why shilajit is free of adverse side effects and is known as the safest dietary supplement. Nevertheless, the astonishing properties of shilajit are entirely due to its chemical makeup. Being stuffed with humic substances, along with more than 84 minerals and metals, shilajit becomes the winner among other natural remedies. Also, the even distribution of these active ingredients ensures that shilajit will never disappoint us and thus, is the safer option   that   provides   enormous   healing   benefits.

CHAPTER #6:
USAGE, DOSAGE, AND SIDE EFFECTS OF SHILAJIT

In ancient times, people were using shilajit in its raw form, directly collected from the mountains. Although it was still providing curative benefits, there was a strong fear of impurities and hazardous chemicals that could deplete the effectiveness of shilajit and may also result in potential side effects. As time passed and people become aware of the harms that come with impure shilajit, they began to formulate methods and techniques to purify the shilajit. Thus, after the discovery of purification methods, shilajit becomes free from impurities and is mixed with additional herbs to further enhance its powers.

FORMS OF SHILAJIT

Now, different forms of shilajit have been introduced and people are using it in different ways according to their needs and tastes. The widely used forms of shilajit are:

1) Solid form

Shilajit is commonly used in the solid form. To get solidified shilajit, shilajit is first converted into resin and then dried several times at high temperatures, either artificially or naturally.

2) Resin

Resin is the purest form of natural shilajit. It has a sticky, tar-like appearance of raw shilajit and is the least purified. That's why resin is high in natural content as compared to other forms of shilajit that have to go through extensive purification methods.

3) Powder form

The powdered form of shilajit is available in black, brown, red, and amber color, and it goes through rigorous purification steps but still, it has more nutritional supply as compared to solid shilajit. Usually, people like shilajit in its powdered form because it is easy to consume and is highly soluble in water, milk, and other drinks.

4) Liquid form

The liquid form is prepared through the evaporation technique and is a more purified version than that of resin shilajit. The liquid shilajit has a thick consistency that can be consumed directly or you can mix it with any drink of your choice.

5) Tablets form

Tablets are recommended for those who don't like other versions of shilajit due to taste, appearance, or any other reason. Tablets have fixed dosages and are in concentrated form.

6) Capsule form

The capsule form contains powdered shilajit inside it and is lower on the nutritional scale as compared to other forms.

HOW TO USE SHILAJIT?

There are different ways to use shilajit and each way is according to its form. Some of the most common forms of shilajit include:

1) Shilajit powder

Shilajit powder can be taken with milk, lukewarm water, tea, smoothies, or any other drink of your choice. Add 2-4 pinches of shilajit to your favorite drink, mix properly, and then drink it twice a day. It would be better if you drink after light meals or in the morning.

2) Shilajit tablets/capsules

Like other tablets, shilajit tablets or capsules can be taken orally with any drink. Take shilajit tablets or capsules two times a day after meals.

3) Resin

Resin can be consumed directly, you can add it to any drink, or prepare syrup of resin by mixing it with a little amount of water. Take resin twice a day, one in the morning to feel energetic throughout the day and the other after any meal.

4) External application of Shilajit

All the above methods are used to get benefits from the shilajit through diet. Another method consists of the external application of shilajit in the form of creams, lotions, and other tonics that have shilajit as their main ingredient. Shilajit is well known for its benefits as an antiaging agent and for promoting healthy and beautiful skin. This is because shilajit contains a number of essential minerals that provide the skin with nourishment and promote skin vitality.

Moreover, you can directly add shilajit to your creams and lotions and apply it to your skin to maximize skin health and appearance. For this, take shilajit and cream base in a ratio of 1:3 and mix them properly. Or you can directly apply shilajit to your skin.

SHILAJIT AND ASHWAGANDHA

The combo of shilajit and ashwagandha is very popular in Indian culture and is often used in ayurvedic medicine.

What is Ashwagandha?

Ashwagandha, also known as Indian ginseng, is a powerful herb that contains bioactive molecules and is packed with amazing health benefits just like shilajit. The medicinal strength of ashwagandha is because of a steroidal molecule called *"Withanolides"*. Withanolide is a potent component that acts as an antistress, reduces anxiety, helps to regulate blood glucose levels, and strengthens the immune system. Ashwagandha is rich in antioxidants, amino acids, fatty acids, alkaloids, and choline and, therefore, is also useful for increasing strength, improving endurance, enhancing cognitive skills, and improving sexual performance.

The combination of Shilajit and Ashwagandha

The combination of shilajit and ashwagandha is very common in ayurvedic medicine. There are many concerns regarding the combined use of both herbs and people often fear that together these potent herbs may cause toxicity and potential harm. But the reality is the opposite. These herbs are powerful rejuvenators and when used together, their strength doubles. For better results, it is recommended to blend these herbs in equal quantities and use them in the method you like. The combined therapy of shilajit and ashwagandha can provide the following health benefits:

- Treats chronic fatigue quickly and more effectively

- Improve sexual performance and increases libido

- Improve physical strength and overall health

- Improve mental health and treat mental disorders

- Extremely beneficial for memory

- Significantly reduces the risk of Alzheimer's

- Best energy booster

- These herbs when combined together, can be used as the most effective treatment for a weak immune system

DOSAGE FOR SHILAJIT

The recommended doses of shilajit dosage are necessary to obtain maximum benefits without causing any potential side effects. There are several factors that will help in determining the exact dosages of shilajit for you. These parameters include:

- Over physical and mental health

- Body mass index (BMI)

- Metabolism

- Weight

- Height

- Lifestyle

- Eating habits

- Age

- Exercise routine or physical activity

In the beginning, you may dislike your experience with the shilajit. You may notice a disturbance in sleeping patterns, problems with the digestive system, and nausea but as time passes, all the discomfort subsides and you will start observing the positive effects of shilajit. In case the discomfort is unbearable or too much disturbing, you are instructed to reduce the dosage of shilajit and increase it gradually until you reach your recommended doses. However, if the symptoms persist then discontinue its use and consult your doctor as soon as possible.

BEST TIME TO TAKE SHILAJIT

The best time for the shilajit is when the absorption rates are higher in the body. The absorption rates are often high and desirable when you take shilajit on an empty stomach in the morning. The second dose should be taken after a light meal preferably before night as taking shilajit at night may disturb your sleeping schedule.

HOW LONG ONE SHOULD CONSUME SHILAJIT?

If you are planning to take shilajit for treatment purposes, then take it as long as your problem persists. After that, stop its use.

However, to gain general health benefits and boost energy, most people consume shilajit throughout their lives.

RECOMMENDED SHILAJIT DOSAGE

It is not possible to prescribe or select the exact recommended dose of shilajit and one has to take the first selected dose continuously for a minimum of 3 days according to the guidelines given above. During the period of 3 days, you should take note of how your body is reacting to shilajit. After 3 days trial period, you can increase or decrease the dose according to your requirements, and if the initial dose suits you then don't change it and stick to it.

Following are the recommended doses for adults, children, pets, and plants.

- **For Adults**

  For adult men and women, the daily recommended dosage of shilajit is 250 to 500 mg twice a day.

- **For Children**

The recommended dosage for children is between 50mg to 100mg. Children are advised to take shilajit only once a day or twice a day depending upon their requirements.

- **For Pets**

You can even use shilajit for your dogs, cats, or other pets. The daily recommended dosage for pets is 50mg but it should be according to the weight and size of the pet. This 50 mg is for pets weighing 150 lbs. Add 50 mg more with every 100lbs and for smaller, randomly reduce the doses according to the pet's weight.

- **For Plants**

Even though shilajit is derived from dead and decomposed plants, it can still add life to other plants and rejuvenate them. The Fulvic content acts as a catalyst or fertilizer for the enzymes present in the soil and these enzymes work in the same way as they function inside the human body. The recommended dose for plants is 150 mg. Mix this recommended amount with a large portion of water and use it two or three times a month.

POTENTIAL SIDE EFFECTS OF SHILAJIT

Although shilajit is the safest herb known and is free of any side effects, in rare cases, shilajit may also result in side effects. These adverse effects often arise due to the use of impure shilajit in its raw form or due to misuse of shilajit, either by consuming too much of it or using it for a long duration. The most commonly observed side effects of shilajit are:

- Burning sensations in feet

- A rise in body temperature

- Increased urination

- Dizziness, Nausea

- Elevated heart rate

- Itching, hives, or other allergic reactions

- Increase level of uric acid

- Toxicity

- There might be a risk of shilajit interaction with other drugs or therapies

PRECAUTIONS

Recommended precautionary measures are:

- Always try to consume a purified form of shilajit

- Get shilajit from trusted sources

- Pregnant and breastfeeding women should consume with great care and only after consulting the expert

- Due to the antidiabetic, antihypertensive, and antidiuretic effects of shilajit, one should take it with proper monitoring of blood pressure and sugar levels

These simple yet important instructions can help you to avoid any potential side effects and you will be able to extract more out of shilajit.

REFERENCES

Agarwal, S. P., Khanna, R., Karmarkar, R., Anwer, M. K., & Khar, R. K. (2007). Shilajit: a review. Phytotherapy Research: An International Journal Devoted to Pharmacological and Toxicological Evaluation of Natural Product Derivatives, 21(5), 401-405.

Biswas, T. K., Pandit, S., Mondal, S., Biswas, S. K., Jana, U., Ghosh, T., ... & Auddy, B. (2010). Clinical evaluation of spermatogenic activity of processed Shilajit in oligospermia. Andrologia, 42(1), 48-56.

Downey, M. Shilajit And Methylene Blue.

Gangwar, S. S., Thakur, R. N., Sharma, R., & Tilak, A. (2016). Shilajit a medicinal mystery to cure the un-cure disease. Imperial J Interdisciplinary Res, 3, 1544-7.

Ghosal, S. (1990). Chemistry of shilajit, an immunomodulatory Ayurvedic rasayan. Pure and Applied Chemistry, 62(7), 1285-1288.

Jadhav, P., & Pagar, H. (2021). Evaluation of Antidepressant activity of Shilajit in experimental animals. Asian Journal of Pharmacology & Toxicology, 9(2), 01-05.

Jadhav, R. P., Kengar, M. D., Narule, O. V., Koli, V. W., & Kumbhar, S. B. (2019). A review on alzheimer's disease (AD) and its herbal treatment of alzheimer's disease. Asian Journal of Research in Pharmaceutical Science, 9(2), 112-122.

Kececi, M., Akpolat, M., Gulle, K., Gencer, E., & Sahbaz, A. (2016). Evaluation of preventive effect of shilajit on radiation-induced apoptosis on ovaries. Archives of gynecology and obstetrics, 293(6), 1255-1262.

Kloskowski, T., Szeliski, K., Krzeszowiak, K., Fekner, Z., Kazimierski, Ł., Jundziłł, A., ... & Pokrywczyńska, M. (2021). Mumio (Shilajit) as a potential chemotherapeutic for the urinary bladder cancer treatment. Scientific Reports, 11(1), 1-12.

Meena, H., Pandey, H. K., Arya, M. C., & Ahmed, Z. (2010). Shilajit: A panacea for high-altitude problems. International journal of Ayurveda research, 1(1), 37.

Pant, K., Singh, B., & Thakur, N. (2012). Shilajit: a humic matter panacea for cancer.

Park, J. S., Kim, G. Y., & Han, K. (2006). The spermatogenic and ovogenic effects of chronically administered Shilajit to rats. Journal of ethnopharmacology, 107(3), 349-353.

Stohs, S. J., Singh, K., Das, A., Roy, S., & Sen, C. K. (2017). Energy and Health Benefits of Shilajit. In Sustained Energy for Enhanced Human Functions and Activity (pp. 187-204). Academic Press.

Trivedi, N. A., Mazumdar, B., Bhatt, J. D., & Hemavathi, K. G. (2004). Effect of shilajit on blood glucose and lipid profile in alloxan-induced diabetic rats. Indian journal of pharmacology, 36(6), 373.

Velmurugan, C., Vivek, B., Wilson, E., Bharathi, T., & Sundaram, T. (2012). Evaluation of safety profile of black shilajit after 91 days repeated administration in rats. Asian Pacific journal of tropical biomedicine, 2(3), 210-214.

Velmurugan, Chinnasamy & Vivek, B. & Shekar, S.B. & Sudha, S.P. & Sundaram, T.. (2010). Shilajit in management of iron deficiency anaemia. J Pharm Biomed Sci. 1. 1-2.

Wilson, E., Rajamanickam, G. V., Dubey, G. P., Klose, P., Musial, F., Saha, F. J., ... & Dobos, G. J. (2011). Review on shilajit used in traditional Indian medicine. Journal of ethnopharmacology, 136(1), 1-9.